KEEP KIDS SAFE

How to Clean and Disinfect
Child-Care Facilities

Produced by Christ Supplies

www.christ-supplies.com

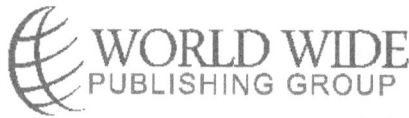

WORLD WIDE
PUBLISHING GROUP

7710-T Cherry Park Dr, Ste 224
Houston, TX 77095
www.WorldwidePublishingGroup.com
(281) 830-8724

The views expressed in this book are the authors and do not necessarily reflect those of the publisher.

Edited by Diane Cottrell, PhD

Cover design by Christian Clark
www.EChristianClark.com

Published in the United States of America.

Ebook: 978-3-9602-8540-3
Softcover: 978-0692477083

Preface

In a child-care setting, apart from loving care, perhaps nothing is more important than to ensure a safe environment. Babies and young children who have yet to develop strong immune systems tend to frequently contract colds and other illnesses due to the fact that they drool, cough, sneeze, and are likely to put anything they touch into their mouths. In addition, they constantly need their diapers changed or assistance at the toilet.

Proper cleaning and disinfecting is required to reduce children's risk of illness caused by bacteria, viruses, mold and fungi. Knowing how to do this is one of the biggest challenges that child-care professionals face. While most of us know that it involves more than hand washing, vacuuming, laundering linens and cleaning toys, fewer of us know that not all cleaning chemicals are safe and appropriate in a child-care setting. For example, the use of common household bleach may be inexpensive, but it can also cause breathing difficulties and corrosive skin burns to small children, as well as trigger an asthma attack for an asthmatic.

Today, more and more "Green" products are being developed as alternatives to those products with harmful chemicals that threaten the health of children, staff and the environment.

The management team of Christ Supplies has decades of experience and a passion for child safety and for Christ, who said "Let the little children come to me, and do not hinder them, for the kingdom of heaven belongs to such as these" (Matthew 19:14). They have compiled this book of information, helpful guidelines and tips from recognized industry experts to assist those responsible for taking care of children in their very important work. They've intentionally kept it brief to encourage you and each of your coworkers to read it and refer to it as needed.

May God bless you and your child-care facility!

Eddie Smith
President/Cofounder, U.S. Prayer Center
Owner/CEO, Worldwide Publishing Group

Table of Contents

Chapter 1

Defining the Issue

Are we all "germophobics" or are our concerns rational and in tune with modern cultural norms? Have you been sick lately? Do you know what caused it? How about friends or loved ones, has anyone you know been sick? Most of us would answer "Yes" to that question.

Have you noticed that antibacterial products seem to be everywhere? The first time I noticed them was a few years ago, when a local hospital installed units by the entrance and encouraged any visitors to sanitize their hands upon entering the facility. Then waste baskets started appearing near the exit doors of most public restrooms. People don't want to touch the door with their washed hands so they carry a paper towel over to the door to open it.

Even supermarkets now have disinfectant wipes available at the entrance for wiping the cart handles. Great idea, except then we go in and handle produce, cans, leaking uncooked meat and poultry, and other food items that have been handled by many people before us. So, what is the answer, and more importantly, is there an answer?

Public officials say "Wash your hands." Great advice, however, most people don't consistently follow this advice. And many don't know the proper techniques for washing their hands. You say "How difficult can that be"? Wash, rinse, dry, and don't touch anything on your way out of the restroom. Maybe your hands are clean, maybe not. Do you know that it takes 15–20 seconds of vigorous washing to effectively remove potentially dangerous pathogens from your hands? Next time you wash your hands, time yourself. I bet you don't make it to 15 seconds. There are too many things to do, too many places to go.

According to the CDC, keeping hands clean is one of the most important things we can do to prevent the transmission of pathogens. People unconsciously touch their eyes, nose, and mouth, transmitting germs from their contaminated hands, thus causing illness. People with contaminated hands also pass these germs onto other surfaces such as doorknobs, handles, rails, etc. that are then touched by other people and the cycle goes on.

Why are we bringing this up? Well, because there are new ideas and new processes and products that can help in reducing the spread of pathogens and the sickness they cause. As we all know, viruses and other pathogens have become part of our daily lives. When that pathogen is Ebola, and it is touted by the news media as a threat to the world population, we all pay attention. But what about the much more common viruses that we meet on an almost daily basis? *Influenza, staph, E. coli, pneumonia, MRSA, norovirus, rotavirus*, and many more are all common in our environment today. Cruise ships and hotels have in recent months been fighting the spread of the *norovirus*. Did you know that this virus can live on a surface up to 6 weeks? Or, that 1,000 particles of this virus can live on the head of a pin? Or, that only 18 particles will make you sick?

Rotavirus spreads easily among infants and young children. They can spread this virus both before and after they have active symptoms. It can be transmitted via contaminated hands and objects such as toys, doorknobs, handles, flush levers, etc. Like influenza, the rotavirus vaccine does not provide full protection from the virus.

We are a high tech, high touch society. Think of all the things you touch during the day, hundreds, maybe thousands of items. If you are a business person, you shake hands often. How many times did the person with whom you just shook hands shake someone else's hand?

You can easily see how the multiplier effect can expose us to thousands of potential pathogens which could cause illness. As these viruses cause illness, thousands of hours of work time are missed. And, a recent study shows that 82% of transmission of viruses is through touch. So, the next time you want to peel off a couple of bills for a tip, and you consider wetting your finger on your tongue, don't. Think about where your hands have been and when you last washed them.

So, who is most susceptible to these viruses? Travelers are one group who are greatly exposed. Millennials aged 18–30 travel more than any other age group, followed by baby boomers aged 46–65. Think of an airport with thousands of people in one building and more and more people coming and going. Do you think this is a haven for pathogens? Notice more and more restrooms have touchless flush systems for their toilets and faucets. But there are so many areas to touch, and the restroom door is one of our greatest enemies.

You have used all the touchless devices in the restroom and washed your hands for 15 seconds, but you still have to exit the restroom. This restroom maybe has no door, which is becoming more prevalent, especially in airports. So you will not touch a door handle or knob. But, you will touch something, and so the cycle continues.

We are adults and should know and follow the proper protocol for sanitation. What about the children? Can you teach them to properly wash their hands or can you even get them to wash their hands? You can at home, but what about the time spent in day care or nursery?

An interesting fact to consider is that, according to the National Institute of Health, 80% of children under the age of 6 spent a mean of 40 hours each week in a child-care setting. In this significant amount of time the child is exposed to many potentially dangerous pathogens.

Let's use influenza as an example. The CDC (Center for Disease Control) states that about 20,000 children less than 5 years of age are hospitalized each year due to complications related to the flu. Child-care centers contribute significantly to the survival of influenza outbreaks. It is worth noting that a child with influenza may be contagious before they even realize they are sick.

In addition, there are several gastrointestinal viruses that are of major concern to infants and young children. Two of the most prevalent are *rotavirus* and *norovirus*. The CDC rates rotavirus as the top cause of diarrhea in infants and young children worldwide. In the U.S., the prevalence of this virus has decreased with the introduction of the rotavirus vaccine. However, neither infection nor immunization provides complete immunity from future infections.

Norovirus is also an extremely contagious virus. It is of special concern for children, since there is no vaccine or specific medication for infections.

Norovirus is often referred to as "stomach flu" or "food poisoning." It causes a condition known as acute gastroenteritis, which is an inflammation of the stomach and/or intestines. This results in stomach pain, diarrhea, nausea, and vomiting. According to the CDC, *norovirus* is the most common cause of acute gastroenteritis in the country causing 19–21 million cases per year. It leads to 1.7–1.9 million office visits and 400,000 emergency room visits per year, primarily in young children. It also results in 56,000 to 71,000 hospitalizations and 570 to 800 deaths, primarily among young children and the elderly population.

Norovirus can be contracted several times in a person's lifetime, as there are several different types of *norovirus*. Becoming ill with one type may not provide immunity from another.

In light of the awareness of the many pathogens which can be easily transmitted, vigilance in preventing outbreaks in child-centered settings is an absolute must. A main component of CDC guidelines for preventing all of the above-mentioned illnesses, as well as so many others, is keeping frequently- touched objects clean and sanitized. Given the limited existence and/or effectiveness of immunizations available for these illnesses, prevention of transmission is clearly the best course of action.

There are many disinfectants and sanitizers on the market today. They differ widely in terms of their safety and the pathogens that they control. Some are more effective than others, some safer in terms of hazards to humans than others.

One widely used disinfectant is chlorine bleach. Although an effective disinfectant, the hazards associated with the use of sodium hypochlorite, the primary ingredient in chlorine bleach, have been well documented. Sodium hypochlorite–based disinfectants should be used judiciously and always with the proper personal protective equipment.

New products and procedures in the marketplace are directed at achieving the CDC's goal of preventing transmission of these pathogens. One example of this is passive germ control technology that is now emerging in a variety of new products.

Passive antimicrobial films are now available as a barrier to protect people from contracting pathogens on surfaces such as children's play elements, doorknobs, faucet handles, and other areas of frequent touch.

Better disinfectants that are more child-friendly are also available. EPA Toxicity Level 4 products, which carry no signal words like Danger, Warning, or Caution on their labels, can be found. Such "Tox 4" products, as they are known, are formulated with less toxic ingredients. They pose a much lower residual health risk to children and are usually more environmentally friendly.

So, it seems apparent that we must do everything possible to minimize the transmission of infectious pathogens, especially for our children and elderly, the most vulnerable classes of our society.

The goal of this publication is to provide information that will enable you to make better decisions regarding products and procedures for cleaning, disinfecting, and maintaining child-care areas.

Chapter 2

Choosing the Right Product

Okay, now you are trying to decide which cleaning chemicals to purchase. But you're not a chemist, and your closest chemist friend is 850 miles away. What to do? (Do 850 miles matter when there's e-mail, let alone cell phones? I would think that it's more likely that a person wouldn't even know a chemist.)

Well, given the right information, this process is not quite as formidable as it might seem. Naturally, you will probably seek advice from your current supplier of cleaning products. That's fine, but recognize that such advice will certainly be somewhat skewed by the particular products that person has available for sale in the product line that they represent.

Generally speaking, no one person has all of the best (or most suitable for your purposes) cleaning products in their arsenal of items to offer you. Furthermore, sales persons themselves may not be as familiar with the fine points of their products as you might expect. In my 40-plus years of experience as a cleaning product formulator, seller, user, and technical service problem-solver, I can't tell you how many problems I have seen which were primarily due to customers using the wrong product for a given purpose. That might have been their fault or the fault of the sales representative. But it does emphasize the critical fact that every cleaning product must be closely matched to the intended end use or frequent application.

Therefore, it behooves you to take the time and effort to become what we'll call "semi-expert" in selecting your products. That is especially important when it comes to products for cleaning and/or disinfecting child-care areas. Children are more vulnerable to undesirable toxic effects from unwanted exposure to residual hazardous chemical ingredients, should they encounter them.

Now becoming "semi-expert" in cleaning products does not require a degree in chemistry. Nor will it be the chore that you might imagine. You'll be surprised at how much information is available and easily obtained when you know where to look for it. And, you may also be surprised to find that a lot of the available information is written for the average person in terminology that most folks can understand. Keeping a dictionary at your elbow is not usually required.

As we all know, this is the age of "Everything on the Internet." Of course it doesn't necessarily follow that all of that information is totally accurate. And you may need to make some comparisons between different sites to arrive at a sound decision. But the Internet is a good place to start. Look for information on best cleaning practices and safest products (from both a health and an environmental perspective).

Check out information and documents from these reliable websites for starters:

CDC Centers for Disease Control
www.cdc.gov

EPA Environmental Protection Agency
www.epa.gov

GC3 Green Chemistry & Commerce Council
www.greenchemistryandcommerce.org

ISSA International Sanitary Supply Association
www.issa.com

NIOSH National Institute for Occupational Safety & Health
www.cdc.gov/niosh

OSHA Occupational Safety and Health Administration
www.osha.gov

With that background, let's get into the matter of **Choosing the Right Product** by stating our objective here. For those tasked with maintaining (including cleaning and disinfecting) child-care areas, we can sum up the overall objective like this:

(1)   Provide a safe play or study environment for the children. Minimize the potential for any injuries.

(2)   As much as possible, utilize products and procedures that reduce the likelihood of pathogenic disease transmission between kids.

(3)   Use cleaning products and procedures that afford the desired results without leaving any undesirable residual product residues that could adversely affect the children.

(4)   Where disinfectants are required, use products that will produce the best results with the least potential for toxic effects on children.

So how to accomplish that? In the following pages of this chapter, we'll provide a list of 20 tips that – if followed – will indeed qualify you as "semi-expert." In fact, you might very well end up smarter than your cleaning chemical sales representative. Our goal in this section is to give you enough tools to choose products with the right chemistry. That means those products that will produce the results you desire without over-buying or over-paying.

Tip #1

NEVER sign a contract with any chemical company, supplier, or distributor. Such contracts only serve to lock you into their products and pricing while locking out the competition. There is no advantage in that for you. If they won't sell to you without a contract, politely tell them "Goodbye." In truth, they will probably agree to serve you without a contract.

Tip #2

Be wary of any arrangement you might be tempted to make that is based upon the supplier providing free products beyond a certain agreed-upon level of usage. Recognize that, if necessary, the supplier will be paying you back with product that costs them a whole lot less than it would cost you.

Tip #3

Start your chemical purchasing process by accurately identifying your product needs. Approach this from the standpoint of clearly evaluating your expectations and communicating those to potential suppliers. You should define the expected results, not the supplier.

Tip #4

If purchasing dispensed chemical products (as for laundry or dish machines), establish a trial period before committing to more extensive purchases.

Tip #5

Decide whether you can utilize environmentally friendly (Green) cleaning products. For the most part, Green products are now as effective as their "Non-Green" counterparts. In a few cases, where especially strong products might be required for certain applications, you may not find a suitable Green replacement. However, for most housekeeping applications, good Green product alternatives are out there. Raw material suppliers have been busy coming up with new Green raw materials, so knowledgeable formulators should be able to take advantage of that. The other thing you should know is that Green cleaning products need not cost you significantly more than comparable Non-Green items. Many Green raw materials have been on the market for some time now, and prices for those raws have come down. So don't overpay for your Green products. Again, it's important to keep the door open to competitive products to ensure that you are purchasing at a fair cost.

In particular, it should be possible to purchase Green products for cleaning all child-care areas. There is no shortage of Green glass cleaners, Green general purpose cleaners, etc. But be careful of certification programs for Green products that are devoid of adequate criteria to back up the Green claim. In our opinion, there are three reliable certification programs for Green cleaning products:

(a)   **EPA DfE** (Design for the Environment; also includes newer **Safer Choice** logo)

(b)   **Green Seal**

(c)   **EcoLogo**

The EPA program is especially robust, with a very extensive set of documents and criteria that a supplier must meet to participate in that program.

Tip #6

Recognize that, in some instances, the quality of your local water supply will dictate product selection. For example, if you have relatively soft water with no iron content, a Green toilet bowl cleaner (if employed with adequate frequency) should be fine. But if your water is hard and/or has a significant level of iron, it will probably be necessary to use an acid-based bowl cleaner. Owing to the acid content, those are not often recognized as Green.

Tip #7

Always obtain Safety Data Sheets (SDS) for all chemical products that you purchase. Those documents used to be called MSDS (Material Safety Data Sheets), but under new global chemical safety regulations the terminology has changed to Safety Data Sheet. Also, the format of the document has been revised to be consistent with international standards. Don't ignore these SDS; they are full of good information on the product. While parts are rather technical, the content is very useful when properly interpreted and applied.

Tip #8

Place all of your chemical product SDS documents in a three-ring binder and place them in a location that is easily accessible to all employees (in the event of an emergency involving a product). Do not put SDS away in a file cabinet. OSHA requires that these Safety Data Sheets can be quickly referenced, if necessary.

Tip #9

Be sure that any chemical product in a spray bottle is clearly marked with an OSHA-approved label for that product. Best to use only spray bottle products in their original containers and then discard the container when empty. Alternatively, spray bottles can be refilled from a suitable dispensing system or a larger container, so long as the bottles have acceptable labels, which should be procured from the suppliers. Merely marking a spray bottle with brief wording like "Glass Cleaner" is not acceptable and could result in a serious fine, if discovered by OSHA.

Tip #10

Did you know that if you have a commercial dish machine (either high-temp or low-temp), it is almost certain that your machine dish detergent is high enough in alkalinity to require a plumbed eyewash station nearby? That is an OSHA regulation that is often (perhaps even usually) ignored. But if, God forbid, you have an employee accident where the machine detergent gets into the employee's eyes, you will likely have a serious problem. The pH of machine dish detergents is usually in the 12–13 range, which means possible permanent eye damage if not quickly rinsed out. Plumbed eyewash stations are not that expensive and certainly worth mitigating the risk. Should you experience that kind of accident, you will definitely not like the fine imposed by OSHA.

Tip #11

Read the label on every chemical product that you have on hand. Moreover, require all of your employees to read and understand those labels as well. Regular employee training is another OSHA requirement, and employee familiarity with product labels is part of that.

Tip #12

If you have multiple products in spray bottles, consider purchasing products with different colors for each different application. The chance of a product being misapplied is lessened when each product is easily distinguishable by color from the others.

Tip #13

So can you easily tell if a chemical cleaning product you are purchasing and using is formulated with the best possible chemical ingredients? Probably not. And even if you were knowledgeable enough to differentiate, it's not that easy. Since most products are formulated with multiple ingredients, it is partly the combination of those ingredients that determines the efficacy (and also the toxicity) of the product. Plus, it is not often possible to make meaningful comparisons between products just for reviewing the product documentation. Nonetheless, the SDS does provide clues. The hazard, first aid, and chemical profile information on the SDS will go a long way toward informing you about what you are dealing with. Should you have questions, or if you are concerned about something on the SDS, ask the supplier for clarification.

Tip #14

Now on to more specific information regarding disinfectants and sanitizers. First, recognize the difference. In the United States, disinfectants and sanitizers (if they make claims to kill anything) are regulated by the Environmental Protection Agency (EPA). Surface disinfectants were previously deemed to kill 100% of pathogenic microorganisms in a specified time. The current EPA requirement is slightly different. It specifies that the surface disinfectant must demonstrate the ability to prevent certain test bacteria from growing in 59 out of 60 samples when left on for a stated dwell time, which can be no more than 10 minutes. Sanitizers are less powerful and usually kill fewer organisms. Sanitizers used on non-food contact surfaces must reduce the number of microbes by at least 99.9% within 5 minutes or less. Sanitizers used on food contact surfaces must reduce the number of microbes by at least 99.999% in 1 minute or less. So don't confuse these two types of antimicrobial products. And don't use the terminology interchangeably. A disinfectant is a disinfectant, and a sanitizer is a sanitizer. They are not the same thing. However, a given concentrated product could be marketed as both a disinfectant and sanitizer. In that case, label directions will clearly stipulate the exact concentration to be used for each application. The disinfectant strength will always be higher.

Tip #15

The difference between the two main types of hard surface sanitizers is referenced above in Tip #14. We probably should also acknowledge that the EPA now recognizes three classifications or levels of disinfecting claims. Each has their own test organisms, and they vary in strength. Without going into more detail, just know that – listed from strongest to weakest – a particular disinfectant could carry a *Healthcare Environment Disinfecting Claim* or a *General or Broad Spectrum Disinfecting Claim* or a *Limited Efficacy Disinfecting Claim*. It would be a good idea to pay some attention to that when deciding what type of disinfectant is appropriate for your intended use.

Tip #16

A disinfectant or sanitizer is not EPA-registered unless the EPA registration number appears on the product label. Also displayed there should be the EPA establishment number, which indicates where the product was manufactured. Always purchase only those disinfectants or sanitizers that contain an EPA registration number. That is your proof that the product has undergone the necessary testing to be approved for its purpose by the EPA. Before marketing a product, the supplier is issued an "EPA Stamped Label" (master label) by the EPA that contains all of the label language approved for that product by the EPA. The supplier does not have to use everything on the EPA Stamped Label, but they cannot use on their product label any language that is not specifically EPA approved and included on the EPA Stamped Approved Label.

Tip #17

That takes us to specific applications for every disinfectant or sanitizer. Never utilize a disinfectant or sanitizer for any purpose or application other than those which are specifically spelled out on the product label. This is very important; the EPA is very picky about it. Basically, if the product in question does not specifically refer to the application you have in mind on its label, you cannot use it for that application. Not all hard surfaces are specifically referenced, however. For example, if a sanitizer is approved for use on hard, non-porous surfaces, then one such surface is deemed to be equivalent to another, regardless of the exact nature of the item. In that sense a stainless steel food prep table would be approved along with the outside surface of an ice machine.

Let's take that rule into the nursery or child-care area. If a disinfectant does not specifically include children's toys in the label directions, it cannot be used for that application. Fortunately, there are EPA-approved disinfectants for those applications – extending all the way down to pacifiers. But check your product label before deciding. Remember, the bottom line is that if the product label or EPA Stamped Approved Label (master label) doesn't state that you can do it, you can't do it. Period.

Tip #18

If you want to know which pathogenic microbes can be killed or reduced by a disinfectant or sanitizer, just refer to the product label. Almost always, the supplier will include every such pathogen on the label. After all, they want to look as good as possible. And testing for effectiveness against each microbe is expensive. So you can be fairly certain that the label reveals everything that the supplier can claim. If the pathogen you are checking for is not listed, then you should not use the product for that application. The key here is the testing process. In reality, the product might be effective against that specific microbe. But if the supplier has not done that efficacy testing, and has not had it submitted to and approved by the EPA, they cannot claim it.

Tip #19

We have talked about Green cleaning products. What about Green disinfectants or sanitizers? Well, here there is not much to offer. Of the three Green certification programs mentioned above in Tip #5, two have made a stab at this. EcoLogo (Canadian-based and now a part of

UL Environment) has certified a few hydrogen peroxide antimicrobial products for Canada. They don't, however, carry the EcoLogo designation in the United States. The EPA, through their DfE program, has approved five active ingredients as eligible for DfE product recognition. Those five ingredients are ethanol, isopropanol, citric acid, L-lactic acid, and hydrogen peroxide. At last count six antimicrobial cleaning products have been authorized to use the EPA DfE logo. All are based on either citric acid or lactic acid. It should be noted, though, that these products usually have more limited efficacy and sometimes longer contact times. Accordingly, it is difficult to recommend them for applications where the aim is to control a more extensive list of pathogenic microorganisms.

Tip #20

Concluding our list of "20 Tips" designed to help you become "semi-expert" in the field of institutional cleaners, disinfectants, and sanitizers, we come to the issue of product toxicity. We'll not deal with toxicity too much here, since this is a lead-in to our next chapter. Chapter 3, written by a prominent toxicologist, will take a more in-depth look at toxicological considerations pertaining to cleaning products and antimicrobials. For now, we will merely point out that EPA-registered antimicrobials fall into one of four classifications, depending upon human toxicity of the product.

Each carries its own signal word on the label, which serves to identify that degree of toxicity. They are:

Category 1	**Danger**
Category 2	**Warning**
Category 3	**Caution**
Category 4	***No signal word***

As is evident, the degree of toxicity declines from Category 1 to Category 4. Consequently, it is prudent to be aware of these classifications when making decisions about disinfectants and sanitizers. Hazard warnings and first-aid recommendations are more stringent for products in Categories 1 and 2. Also, the absence of any signal word for Category 4 products means that these products pose the lowest health threat. In fact, ingredients in Category 4 products are usually found on the U.S. Government list of GRAS (Generally Recognized As Safe) ingredients. As such, Tox Category 4 products should be particularly well suited for use in child-care and day care areas.

Chapter 3
Toxicological Considerations

Introduction

This chapter is designed to explain basic concepts associated with the toxicity of different types of cleaners, and to inform your selection of specific cleaners. A trip down the cleaning products aisle at a Costco, Home Depot, or Walmart is overwhelming, with literally hundreds of cleaning products to choose from in liquid, aerosol, powdered, and concentrated form. Many cleaning products currently marketed still contain old ingredient mainstays that your grandparents used to clean at the turn of the century. For example, acetic acid (better known as vinegar) has been used for hundreds of years, sodium hypochlorite (bleach) made its debut in 1914 and was ultimately named Clorox® liquid bleach, and Pine-Sol® disinfectant and deodorizer was invented in 1929 by chemist Harry A. Cole. Many of these early cleaning ingredients were selected because they could clean well, with safety an afterthought.

Understanding the harm that cleaning products can cause can help you use such products safely (by wearing gloves or protective clothing to minimize dermal exposure, or ensuring that there is adequate ventilation to minimize inhalation exposure during use of a cleaning product), as well as inform selection of appropriate cleaners to accomplish the type of cleaning required for specific scenarios (e.g., selecting a sanitizer over a disinfectant if simple sanitization is required). According to the U.S. Centers for Disease Control and Prevention (CDC), the misuse of cleaning products harms both children and adults.[1] The CDC reports most common causes of poisoning among young children are due to misuse of cosmetics and personal care products, household cleaning products, and pain relievers.

Common causes of poisoning among adults are pain relievers, prescription drugs, sedatives, cleaning products, and antidepressants.

A Toxicologist's Perspective

Toxicologists are scientists who work to assess the dangers of chemical and microbiological substances, and ideally, toxicologists seek to reduce those hazards by identifying safer substitutes or finding ways to eliminate the need for hazardous substances in formulations.

---

[1] http://www.cdc.gov/healthyhomes/bytopic/poisoning.html

Toxicologists who assess the safety of cleaning products are often asked the question, "Why is it important to understand human health and environmental risks of using general purpose cleaners, sanitizers, and disinfectants?" A 1967 Christmas Eve sermon from Dr. Martin Luther King answers this question perfectly:

"It really boils down to this: that all life is interrelated. We are all caught in an inescapable network of mutuality, tied into a single garment of destiny. Whatever affects one destiny, affects all indirectly." –Dr. Martin Luther King

By nature of their intended use to kill microorganisms, sanitizers and disinfectants can be quite toxic to humans because they are formulated to cause toxicity to pathogenic microorganisms as part of the cleaning process. While general purpose cleaning products do not kill microorganisms, some ingredients in general purpose cleaners also have toxicity concerns, and may injure skin or eyes, or cause illness or death if the product is misused. Chemicals in general purpose cleaning, sanitizing, and disinfecting products may cause harm to our health or to the environment.

Overview of Health Effects from Exposure to Toxic Chemicals in Cleaning Products

Chemicals in cleaning products impact our health as we inhale these chemicals, absorb them through our skin, or accidentally splash them in our eyes. Young children and unborn children are particularly sensitive to toxic chemicals. For one thing, children consume more air and food relative to their body size compared to adults. The same is true of the amount of skin covering children's bodies – that is, children have a greater dermal surface area relative to their body weight compared to adults. This means that children are particularly susceptible to the harmful effects of chemicals as exposure occurs and are less able to get rid of toxic substances from their bodies than adults. Children are also at risk of greater exposure to chemicals, particularly in child-care environments, due to certain behaviors such as crawling and frequently mouthing objects, which may contain chemical residues on surfaces, or in dust.

A toxicologist can predict the short- and long-term toxicity of chemicals in cleaning products by answering the following questions. How and where on your body are you exposed to the cleaning product? How long does the exposure occur? How much of the cleaning product are you exposed to? How hazardous or toxic are the chemicals used in the cleaning product?

Immediate impacts to our health are called *acute effects* and long-term impacts to our health are called *chronic effects*. Overexposure to cleaning products can cause both acute and chronic adverse health effects. Acute and chronic health effects are described in detail below.

Acute Health Effects

Acute health effects occur over a short period of time. Acute health effects result from either a single exposure to a hazardous chemical or multiple exposures in a short period of time. Examples of acute health effects include asthma, skin and eye irritation and/or corrosion, and allergic reactions on the skin.

Asthma is an inflammatory disease of the lungs and airways, causing passages to become inflamed and narrow, making it very difficult to breathe. An asthma-like response can be caused by a single incident of exposure to a very irritating chemical, which is called Reactive Airways Dysfunction Syndrome (RADS). Skin irritation is a localized, reversible redness, swelling, or damage to the skin resulting from exposure to a substance, while skin corrosion (also known as skin burns) involves permanent damage to the skin and underlying tissue. Eye irritation is a localized, reversible damage to the eye surface resulting from exposure to a substance. In contrast, eye corrosion is a condition that can be described as tissue damage on the eye, or serious physical decay of vision, that does not reverse after 21 days of exposure. Skin sensitization is an allergic response to a substance, and is better known as allergic contact dermatitis (ACD). Allergic contact dermatitis occurs in two phases: first, skin reacts to an exposure to an allergen and this exposure primes the immune system to become sensitized to that allergen, and later, when the skin is exposed to the allergen again, the immune system launches an aggressive inflammatory response that results in itching, bumps, and redness on the skin.

Identifying Categories of Acute Toxicity

Disinfectants and sanitizers are regulated as pesticides by the U.S. Environmental Protection Agency. A pesticide is any substance or mixture of substances intended to prevent, destroy, repel, or mitigate any pest. This definition is broad and pathogenic microorganisms are not typically thought of as "pests," but ingredients with "antimicrobial" properties are intended to destroy microorganisms such as bacteria, mold, and viruses, and the U.S. EPA considers these microorganisms to be pests.

The EPA assesses the toxicity of registered antimicrobials and assigns a precautionary statement for each registered antimicrobial product so that people who use these products may recognize the danger associated with misuse of the product. These precautionary statements are assigned based on hazard classifications of the pesticide ingredients used in cleaning products (known as "actives"), although there are additional "inert" ingredients such as solvents in the products that do not fall under these labeling requirements U.S. EPA's precautionary statements decrease in their degree of toxicity (from highest to lowest health hazard):[2]

- **Category I: Danger**
  - o "Danger" on a label for a pesticide product means that the pesticide product is highly toxic by at least one route of exposure. It may be corrosive, causing irreversible damage to the skin or eyes. Alternatively, it may be highly toxic if eaten, absorbed through the skin, or inhaled (if this is the case, "poison" and the skull and crossbones symbol ☠ must appear on the label).

- **Category II: Warning**
  - o "Warning" on a label for a pesticide product means that pesticide product is moderately toxic if eaten, absorbed through

_____

[2] For more information, please see
http://www2.epa.gov/sites/production/files/2014-07/documents/chapter7_revised_final_0714.pdf
and
http://www.npic.orst.edu/factsheets/signalwords.pdf

the skin, or inhaled, or if it causes moderate eye or skin irritation.

- **Category III: Caution**
  - o "Caution" on a label for a pesticide product means that the pesticide product is slightly toxic if eaten, absorbed through the skin, inhaled, or if it causes slight eye or skin irritation.

- **Category IV: No signal word**
  - o This means that the pesticide product is likely to cause very low toxicity following exposure.

These hazard classifications and their associated precautionary statements provide information about the toxicity, irritation, and sensitization hazards associated with the use of an antimicrobial. In effect, they inform us of the acute health effects associated with a cleaning product containing a registered pesticide.

Systemic toxicity refers to adverse effects that occur as a toxicant is absorbed and is distributed throughout the body, causing harm at a site different than the point of entry of that toxicant. Oral exposure occurs when a chemical is ingested. Dermal exposure occurs when a cleaning product comes into contact with skin. Inhalation exposure occurs by breathing in the fumes of a chemical. Some chemicals in cleaning products (such as isopropyl alcohol or dipropylene glycol monomethyl ether) are very volatile, and move quickly from a cleaning product into the air, and then may be inhaled as the product is used.

Eye and skin irritation and corrosion studies measure irritation or corrosion to the eyes and skin, respectively. Finally, registration of an antimicrobial pesticide also requires a dermal sensitization test to evaluate the potential for the antimicrobial to cause allergic contact dermatitis. However, dermal sensitization results are not assigned to an EPA toxicity category. Based on the results of the five primary acute toxicity studies, a product is assigned a category classification and associated precautionary statements for each effect. For example, a product that contains an ingredient assigned the classification of Category 1 for acute oral toxicity would be labeled with the precautionary statement "Fatal if swallowed" (see Figure 1, below).

Chronic Health Effects

Chronic health effects result from repeated exposures to a chemical over a long period of time or from chemicals that are stored in our bodies. Adverse effects from chronic exposure to a chemical may take months or many years to develop. As such, these chronic effects are not well understood; it can be difficult to associate the development of a disease with an exposure to a specific hazardous chemical that occurred long before the disease developed. Unlike acute effects, there is no parallel classification system and labeling system for chronic effects of ingredients in cleaning products. As detailed below, chronic health effects include asthma, reproductive and developmental toxicity, cancer, and endocrine disruption.

Although asthma can result from a single, concentrated exposure to an irritating chemical, asthma can also develop over time in somebody who has never had asthma before. Asthma may develop through small exposures to a sensitizing chemical over time, which causes the immune system to react more and more strongly as each exposure occurs. Once asthma develops, many triggers, including irritating chemicals, can elicit an asthma attack. The California Department of Public Health found that the rate of work-related asthma among janitors and cleaners is nearly double the rate in the overall workforce. Nationally, in states that keep track of work-related asthma (WRA), 12% of all confirmed cases of WRA are associated with cleaning products.[3]

Reproductive toxicants interfere with normal reproduction, for example by affecting fertility, and cause developmental toxicity which interferes with development of the offspring before and after birth. Chemicals that cause endocrine disruption interrupt or

---

[3] http://www.cdph.ca.gov/programs/IAQ/Pages/CleaningProducts.aspx

imitate the natural hormonal messages in our body that regulate normal functioning.

As young children and unborn children are still developing, early life exposure to toxic chemicals that can cause chronic health effects is particularly troublesome. Because chronic effects, including those that impact development, are not well understood, it is even more important to limit the exposure of young children to hazardous chemicals.

Table 1 presents chemicals often found in cleaning products, and their associated acute, chronic, and environmental toxicity concerns.

Table 1: Chemicals in Cleaning Products that Pose Hazards to Human Health and/or the Environment

Chemical	Uses	Adverse Effects
Ammonia	Solvent	• Acute effects: o Acute inhalation toxicity o Skin irritation o Eye irritation o Respiratory irritation • Chronic effects: o Genotoxicity o Irritant-induced respiratory sensitization • Environmental effects: o Aquatic toxicity

Chlorine Bleach	Antimicrobial	• Acute effects o Skin irritation o Eye irritation o Respiratory tract irritation • Chronic effects o Asthma
Ortho-Phenylphenol	Antimicrobial	• Chronic effects o Cancer
Quaternary Ammonium compounds (e.g., alkyl dimethyl benzyl ammonium chloride & didecyl dimethyl benzyl ammonium chloride)	Antimicrobial, Surfactants	• Acute effects o Skin irritation o Eye irritation o Respiratory tract irritation, asthma • Chronic effects o Developmental toxicity • Environmental effects o Persistent in environment o Toxic to aquatic organisms (e.g., fish)
Fragrance ingredients (up to 3,000 separate chemicals)	Provides scents in cleaning products	• Acute effects o Asthma o Allergic contact dermatitis • Chronic effects o Reproductive toxicity o Cancer • Environmental effects o Persistent in environment o Toxic to aquatic organisms (e.g., fish) o Bioaccumulation

Triclosan	Antibacterial	• Acute effects ○ Skin irritation ○ Eye irritation • Chronic effects ○ Suspected endocrine disruption • Environmental effects ○ Persistent in environment ○ Toxic to aquatic organisms (e.g., fish) ○ Bioaccumulation

Hazard Labelling of Cleaning Products

Understanding hazard classifications and precaution-nary statements associated with U.S. EPA-registered antimicrobial cleaners and general purpose cleaners can guide purchasing decisions and proper use of products and safety precautions (e.g., be careful to keep products labeled with "Danger" out of reach of children who may unknowingly ingest them).

Labelling on general purpose cleaners that don't contain pesticidal ingredients is regulated by the U.S. Federal Hazardous Substance Act (FHSA) regulations, which restrict the use of certain hazardous substances in consumer products and require hazard labeling on consumer products containing hazardous substances. Required product labels also provide information regarding how to protect the consumer and their children from potential hazards, storage information for the product, and first-aid measures if an accident occurs. Under the FHSA, certain products may be banned if the labeling requirements are not adequate to protect the consumer from the hazards of the product.

In contrast, registered sanitizers and disinfectants in the United States must be labelled following rules established by the U.S. EPA. How does the EPA assess the acute human toxicity of registered sanitizers and disinfectants and determine precautionary statements on labeling that belong on each product? The classifications and precautionary statements are based on the results of five hazard tests:

- Acute oral toxicity
- Acute dermal toxicity
- Acute inhalation toxicity
- Eye irritation
- Skin irritation

The acute oral, dermal, and inhalation toxicity tests assess localized and systemic toxicity of a formulation based on the designated route of exposure. Based on the results of the five primary acute toxicity studies, a pesticide-containing product is assigned an EPA category classification, and the EPA requires associated precautionary statements on the label for each effect. Note that while no signal word is associated with dermal sensitization, products that test positive for dermal sensitization (i.e., causing skin allergies) may be required to bear precautionary label language for this endpoint such as: "Prolonged or frequently repeated skin contact may cause allergic reactions in some individuals."

As shown in Figure 1, the skull and crossbones symbol on a cleaning product indicates the product is fatal or toxic and should be used with care and should always be safely stored out of reach of children.

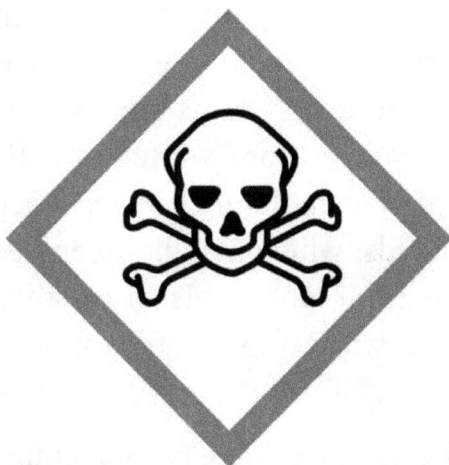

Figure 1: Skull & Crossbones Symbol on a Hazardous Cleaning Product

Overview of Environmental Effects from Exposure to Hazardous Chemicals in Cleaning Products

Up to this point, this chapter has covered how hazardous ingredients in cleaning, sanitizing, and disinfecting products harm our health; however, these ingredients can be hazardous to the environment as well. For example, when a sanitizing product is applied to a countertop and is later rinsed, the rinse water is disposed of down the drain. That wastewater travels down the drain and into a municipal wastewater or a septic system. Wastewater treatment systems are not able to remove all hazardous chemicals from wastewater. Similarly, septic systems in rural communities release septic water into septic drain fields, which may pollute underground water supplies. Therefore, chemicals in cleaning products end up back in our water supply and can pollute air, water, and soil.

A typical example of an environmental toxic chemical in cleaning products is the antimicrobial Triclosan, which is commonly added to hand soaps and hand wipes. The Canadian Environmental Law Association (CELA) found that 95% of the human use of Triclosan goes down the drain and is highly toxic in the aquatic environment, particularly to fish and other aquatic species, persistent, and bioaccumulative, and is present in wastewater treatment plant effluents as well as in sewage sludge.[4]

---

[4] http://www.cela.ca/triclosan-and-triclocarban and

Another example of an environmentally toxic chemical is the chemical nonyl phenol, which is a byproduct of a class of chemicals known as nonylphenol ethoxylates (NPEs). NPEs are used in detergents and cleaning products, and are somewhat notorious because they become *more* toxic as they degrade! Exposure to NPE metabolites causes aquatic organisms to develop both male and female sex organs. Although the use of NPEs in cleaning products such as detergents continues to decline because of legislation (e.g., NPEs cannot be used in detergents sold in the European Union), NPEs still manage to get into the environment, despite their known hazards of these compounds.[5]

These chemicals can harm aquatic organisms, much as they cause harm to humans who are exposed. In some cases, these chemicals break down very slowly and persist in the environment for a very long time. These chemicals end up in aquatic wildlife and build up in the supply chain as smaller organisms are eaten by larger organisms, a process called bioaccumulation. This also means they may end up back in humans as we consume aquatic wildlife.

In the United States, there is no labeling requirement for chemicals in cleaning products that pose environmental hazards, but it is important to be aware of the environmental impacts of chemicals used to clean in

---

http://www.cela.ca/sites/cela.ca/files/triclosan_statement.pdf
[5] http://www2.epa.gov/saferchoice/partnership-evaluate-alternatives-nonylphenol-ethoxylates

order to select cleaning products that are safe for both humans as well as wildlife.

Reducing Health and Environmental Hazards from Cleaning Products

Using cleaning products properly and purchasing less hazardous cleaners, sanitizers, and disinfectants can reduce harmful human health and environmental impacts. A common misconception among consumers is that disinfectants are always the best choice to ensure that surfaces and objects are clean. However, disinfectants aren't always the best choice for cleaning because they don't always remove grime and dirt, thus allowing microorganisms to hide and avoid removal from a dirty surface or object.

Proper Use of Cleaning Products

Harmful exposures to toxic chemicals can also depend on the product's physical characteristics as well as the characteristics of the environment it is used in. Therefore, using the product only in the manner directed on the label is important, because improper use can increase exposure to hazardous chemical ingredients in a cleaning product. Also, knowing when it is appropriate to use a sanitizer (e.g., reducing target microorganisms by 99.9% on non-food, hard surfaces or 99.999% on food surfaces) instead of a disinfectant (reducing 99.999% of target microorganisms on all surfaces) can reduce exposure to toxic chemicals, as disinfectants are stronger and have higher concentrations of active ingredients.

An aerosolized product with instructions to be used in a well-ventilated area should never be used in an enclosed environment; using the product in an enclosed environment with poor ventilation may increase inhalation exposure to the active chemicals in the product. In addition, diluting concentrated products properly is important to ensure the correct amount of a given chemical is used in the final product.

Household bleach has been used for decades as a disinfectant, but should never be mixed with other chemicals, such as ammonia and acids. Ammonia is commonly found in cleaning product such as glass and window cleaners. Mixing bleach and ammonia produces a toxic gas called chloramine, which can result in irritation to the respiratory system and even pneumonia. Acids, including household vinegar, are frequently found in some glass, window, toilet bowl, and drain cleaners. Mixing bleach and acids releases chlorine gas into the air which can cause severe irritation and, in very high levels, even death.

Purchasing Safer Cleaning Products

Using less hazardous cleaning and antimicrobial products can reduce the health and environmental impacts of using such products, particularly for children. There are three primary programs in North America that certify safer cleaning products: U.S. EPA Safer Choice (formerly the Design for the Environment [DfE] Program), GreenSeal, and Ecologo. All three programs strive to recognize cleaning product formulations that are safest in their class and minimize harm to humans and ecosystems. Because pesticidal formulations must be registered with the EPA in the United States, only EPA may recognize "safer" antimicrobial cleaning products in the United States. U.S. EPA's Design for the Environment (DfE) Antimicrobial Pesticide Pilot Program's goal is to move towards the green end of the pesticide spectrum, and make it easy for you to identify "safer" antimicrobial products.[6] U.S. EPA has identified

---

[6] http://www.epa.gov/pesticides/regulating/labels/design-dfe-pilot.html

seven active ingredients that may be used in antimicrobial pesticide products that can be part of the DfE Antimicrobial Pilot Program:

- Citric acid
- Hydrogen peroxide
- L-lactic acid
- Ethanol
- Isopropanol
- Peroxyacetic acid
- Tetraacetylethylenediamine (TAED)

As part of participating in the U.S. EPA DfE Antimicrobial Pilot Program, antimicrobial products and their inert ingredients are also reviewed against EPA's Safer Choice Standard (http://www2.epa.gov/saferchoice/standard). Compliance with the U.S. EPA Safer Choice Standard ensures that the product is not persistent, bioaccumulative, or aquatically toxic. Finding the U.S. EPA Design for the Environment logo on an antimicrobial pesticide product indicates:

It is a Category 3 or Category 4 with respect to EPA's acute hazard classifications. That means the product carries a slight to low health hazard. Specifically, the product:

- Is unlikely to cause chronic health effects, such as:
  - cancer
  - endocrine disruption
  - developmental, reproductive, muta-genic, or neurotoxicity issues
- Is in compliance with U.S. EPA data requirements
- Ingredients have all been reviewed and accepted by U.S. EPA
- Does not require use of mandated personal protective equipment
- Has no unresolved or unreasonable adverse effects
- Has no unresolved performance issues

Participation in the certification programs shown in Figure 2 also ensures that a full ingredient list is available on the label for review, even though regulatory requirements only require the labeling of active ingredients (i.e., antimicrobials).

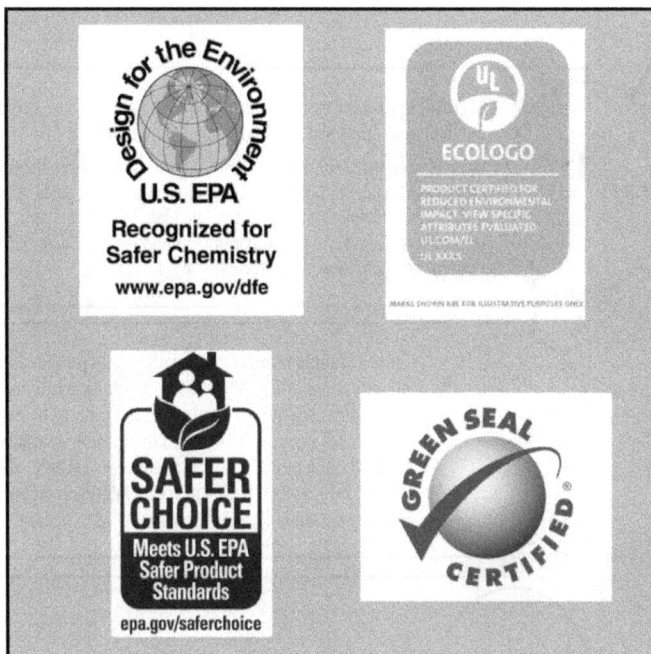

Figure 2: Logos for Third-party Certified Cleaning Products

Using less hazardous cleaning, sanitizing, and disinfecting products will protect the health of those using the products as well as children who use the space, and will also be better for the environment. We have provided tips for finding safer cleaning products below in Figure 3, and tips for finding safer disinfectants and sanitizers in Figure 4.

Tip #1

Look for third-party certifications: U.S. EPA Safer Choice, Ecologo, and GreenSeal are great starts to find safer cleaning products.

Even if a product does not carry a third-party certification, there are several steps you can take to purchase safer cleaning products, particularly by reviewing guidelines for cleaning product labeling. (https://www.issa.com/data/moxiestorage/regulatory_education/regulatory-reference-library/consumer_precautionary_label.pdf).

Tip #2

Some cleaning products have voluntarily provided full ingredient lists on their products. Look for a full ingredient list and avoid certain ingredients (like those listed in Table 1). Some other ingredients to avoid in cleaning products due to human health or environmental concerns include: Bisphenol A (BPA), d-limonene, parabens, phthalates, and ethanolamines (e.g., monoethanolamine, diethanolamine, triethanolamine).

Tip #3

Avoid aerosolized cleaning products, which make chemicals readily available in the air we breathe.

Tip #4

Look for cleaning products which are fragrance-free and dye-free; neither is necessary for the function of the product. However, "unscented" does not mean the same thing as "fragrance-free." Dyes are easily identified with "FD&C" or "D&C" before the name of the colorant.

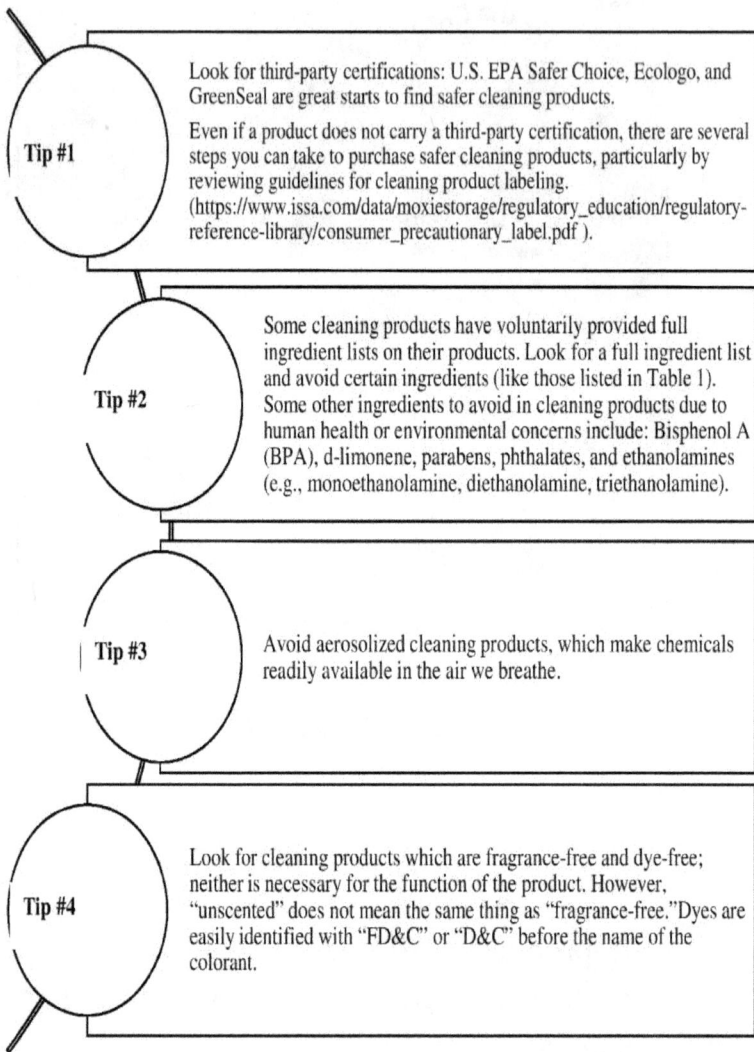

Figure 3: Tips for Finding Safer Cleaning Products

Tip #1

When searching for safer sanitizers and disinfectants, look for the U.S. EPA Design for the Environment (DfE) logo on the product label. The list of sanitizers and disinfectants currently participating in the DfE program can be found at: http://www.epa.gov/pesticides/regulating/labels/design-dfe-pilot.html

Tip #2

Select disinfectants that feature **No** signal word or the signal word **Caution** <u>instead</u> of the signal word **Warning** or **Danger** on the product label. As explained earlier in this chapter, U.S. EPA's four classifications for the acute hazards of pesticide products address short-term toxicity. Therefore, using products which carry labels indicating lower toxicity, such as Category 3 "Caution" and Category 4 "No signal word," helps avoid chemicals with acute hazardous effects.

Figure 4: Tips for Finding Safer Sanitizers and Disinfectants

CONCLUSION

This chapter has been written to communicate the importance of selecting safer cleaning products from both a human health and environmental point of view. There are literally thousands of cleaning products available to clean, polish, scour, shine, sanitize, and/or disinfect surfaces and objects with which we come into contact. Following tips recommended in this chapter is relatively easy and is a positive way to contribute to the world (and much quicker to do than the years of study needed to become a toxicologist!).

By selecting safer cleaning products, you will directly improve the health of cleaning professionals who use these products, children and adults who are exposed to chemicals on surfaces and objects that have come into contact with these products, and countless creatures who share the earth with us. Such actions exemplify the words quoted earlier in this chapter from Dr. King, and contribute to a world we are not ashamed to leave to future generations.

Chapter 4

The Advantages and Disadvantages of Product Certifications [7]

There are tens of thousands of chemicals in commerce in the United States. Many chemicals may have a range of negative impacts on health, the environment, and the economy during their life cycle, from manufacture, through use and disposal. It should be a key part of any sustainable purchasing program to understand which of these chemicals could pose hazards in products and services procured, how they might harm users of those products or the environment, and what safer alternatives are on the market. Institutional purchasers are in a unique position to shift the marketplace towards safer, more sustainable, and more effective cleaning and disinfecting products. And there are many examples of such efforts. However, purchasers generally do not have the technical knowledge, access to information, or time to weigh complex toxicological information to make an informed

---

[7] Adapted from: Perlmutter, A. 2015. Advancing Safer Chemicals in Products: The Key Role of Purchasing. Lowell Center for Sustainable Production, University of Massachusetts Lowell. Accessible at: http://saferalternatives.org//assets/media/documents/uml-rpt-greenpurchasing-715-web.pdf

decision. Price and performance tend to dominate such purchasing decisions.

To address these challenges and simplify the purchasing of more sustainable products, many organizations are requiring the purchase of products that have obtained a particular sustainability certification or certifications. A certification is given to a product by a third party to attest that it meets standards or criteria specified by that third party. Sustainability-related certifications, often demarcated by an Ecolabel,[8] can help purchasers and their suppliers to determine which products are safer for human health and the environment. Requiring the purchase of products that conform to the requirements of these certifications saves purchasers the work of sorting through the various claims and data for individual products and having to become sustainability experts; purchasers only need to learn what types of products the certification covers and what criteria it includes in order to determine which certifications to specify and require that the products purchased conform to the selected standards.

These certification programs make the purchase of lower-toxicity products much easier because they level the playing field among products and ensure that the supplier's claims are verified. Specifying that products meet certain certifications can also prevent bid challenges because the selection criteria are more transparent and

---

[8] Global Ecolabelling Network, What is Ecolabelling, http://www.globalecolabelling.net/what_is_ecolabelling/index.htm

defensible. Certifications currently exist that are publicly and privately sponsored.

Participating in certification programs is also helpful to manufacturers and suppliers. It makes it easier for both groups to identify products they offer that meet widely accepted environmental standards and criteria. In addition, it can reduce the need for them to fill out separate disclosure forms and comply with varying environmental requirements from each organization that wants to purchase their products. Finally, it helps them build their products or offerings to one (or a small) set of environmental requirements rather than to the different requirements of every purchasing organization, and demonstrating product conformance to certifying entities helps suppliers maintain the security of their confidential business information.

However, there are cautions and limits to relying on certifications, and these should be understood by those wanting to buy safer products, since not all of standards and certifications are created equal. It is important for purchasers to understand the certifications that they are considering to ensure that the products meet the criteria that are important to them and to accomplishing their purchasing goals.

For example, certifications might not exist for certain products or categories of products. Some certifications, moreover, only cover a single low-toxicity chemical (such as formaldehyde) or attribute (low Volatile Organic Compound, VOC). These are more limited than multi-attribute certifications such as <u>Green Seal</u>,[9] <u>Cradle to Cradle</u>,[10] <u>Ecologo</u>,[11] and <u>Safer Choice</u>[12] that screen out many chemicals or classes of chemicals, and include in their standard criteria the addressing of a fuller range of other environmental and health endpoints, such as recycled content, use of renewable materials, and more.

Some certifications look at the entire product lifecycle (manufacture, use, and disposal), while others only look at a specific part of it, such as product use or disposal. Some only give points or credit to products that meet certain low-toxicity criteria—but don't include that as a mandatory requirement.

Some certifications—particularly those that are developed solely by product manufacturers, distributors, or industry trade associations—may claim, often with little or no transparent information to back up the claim, that products are safer or less toxic; these could be a type of "<u>greenwashing</u>"[13]. Other certifications can be viewed as relatively weak if the criteria they are based on are not transparent, evenly applied, or rigorous compared to other competing ecolabels in the same category.

---

[9] http://www.greenseal.org/

[10] http://www.c2ccertified.org/

[11] Underwriters Laboratories, Ecologo Product Certification, http://industries.ul.com/environment/certificationvalidation-marks/ecologo-product-certification

[12] http://www2.epa.gov/saferchoice

[13] Underwriters Laboratories, The Sins of Greenwashing, http://sinsofgreenwashing.com/findings/the-seven-sins/

Certain certifications may also be misleading if not properly understood. For example, products such as furniture and paint that have been awarded an ecolabel indicating that they are "low-emitting" may still contain chemicals of concern. While these "low-emitting" products are certified to release lower amounts of formaldehyde or other harmful chemicals, they may still cause harm to users over time, as well as toxic chemical-pollution problems from product manufacturing and disposal.

The most credible certifications are made by an accredited (by a member of the International Accreditation Forum[14] to ISO 17065[15] or ISO 17020[16] standards) independent third party. The standards should be clear and publicly available, and include criteria that require the review of lab results provided by the manufacturer, assessment of the chemical ingredients to ensure that they are safe both individually and in combination, and auditing of the manufacturing process. Some of the certification programs, such as EPA's Safer Choice[17], have made it a requirement that products

---

[14] http://www.iaf.nu/

[15] ISO, Conformity assessment -- Requirements for bodies certifying products, processes and services, ISO/IEC 17065:2012, http://www.iso.org/iso/catalogue_detail.htm?csnumber=46568

[16] ISO, Conformity assessment -- Requirements for the operation of various types of bodies performing inspection, ISO/IEC 17020:2012, http://www.iso.org/iso/catalogue_detail?csnumber=52994

[17] http://www2.epa.gov/saferchoice

carrying their label must disclose the types of ingredients they contain.

Just because a product does not carry an ecolabel does not mean it is toxic or bad for the environment. There may be safer, high performing products on the market that have not gone through a certification process, or a certification may not yet exist for that type of product or may be so new that few products have received it. Manufacturers may choose not to have their products go through the certification process due to the time or expense the process takes. Purchasers can make the effort and expense pay off by using their contracts to reward companies that have gone to the trouble to get their products certified by an independent third party.

While requiring a certification is an important first step in purchasing more sustainable products, deferring to certifications lets the standard's developer, in essence, determine for the purchasing organization what "green" is, instead of leaving it to the purchasing organization to set clear priorities based on its own needs and interests and the potential ways its workers and customers might be exposed. In such cases, where certifications do exist to cover the desired products, purchasers can use them as a starting point and add additional chemical restrictions if they want even stronger standards to be applied.

The U.S. Environmental Protection Agency (EPA) has established a <u>Safer Products Portal</u>[18] that contains information about ecolabels and standards. EPA also recently issued <u>draft guidance</u>[19] to ensure the quality and usability of non-governmental standards and ecolabels for federal procurement efforts; this may be useful for other purchasing professionals and for those setting purchasing policies. A list of some of the more common credible ecolabels are described in the Tools and Resource Section of this document. The Responsible Purchasing Network has also published a list of credible third-party labels.[20]

Regardless of whether or not one specifies a product with a sustainability certification, it is still important to have a system in place to verify that chemicals of concern to the purchasing organization are addressed by the underlying standard, and that any products not covered by a certification exclude these substances.

---

[18] US EPA, Greener Products, Introduction to Eco-Labels and Standards, http://www.epa.gov/greenerproducts/standards/index.html

[19] US EPA, Draft Guidelines for Product Environmental Performance Standards and Ecolabels for Voluntary Use in Federal Procurement, March 2015, http://www.epa.gov/epp/draftGuidelines/

[20] http://www.responsiblepurchasing.org/purchasing_guides/all/standards/

Chapter 5

How to Avoid Problems

Introduction

This chapter focuses on the critical role that an effective cleaning and hand hygiene program plays in protecting public health by preventing the transmission of infectious diseases—from the common cold and flu, to the more exotic *norovirus* and *Methicillin-Resistant Staphylococcus Aureus (MRSA)*.

Each year, infectious diseases such as seasonal influenza exact a substantial toll on society in terms of economic and social losses, as well as human pain and suffering, impacting schools, nurseries, churches, and other places that the general public gathers. Likewise, the common cold is the main reason children miss school and adults miss work, literally affecting millions of individuals annually. Yet, the solution to preventing the spread of these and other infectious diseases is often overlooked—effective cleaning and hand hygiene.

An effective cleaning and hand hygiene program can substantially reduce the spread of influenza, the cold, *norovirus, MRSA* and other infectious diseases, and likewise reduce the health, social, and economic costs associated with these illnesses. In effect, a modest investment in an effective cleaning regimen provides a valuable return in terms of improved human health, enhanced quality of the indoor environment, reduced absenteeism, and increased productivity.

This chapter focuses on the critical role cleaning plays in preventing the transmission of infectious diseases, and provides recommendations and resources that empower facilities to implement a highly effective cleaning regimen that will reduce risks to human health and otherwise contribute to a healthy and productive indoor environment.

Health and Economic Drivers

Progressive churches, day care centers, nurseries, and other such facilities are increasingly adopting a more holistic approach toward protecting the health and well-being of children and other occupants of those facilities through effective cleaning and hand hygiene. That is because research has proven that relatively small incremental investments in cleaning produces substantial benefits in terms of the quality of the indoor environment and improved health and productivity.

Illnesses such as colds, flu, stomach upsets, and headaches are the most common cause of student absences, and have a substantial social and economic cost. Consider the common cold, which results in no less than 22 million missed days of school per year, and an estimated 20 million absences from work due in large part to the need to take time off to care for sick children. All of this results in an estimated total annual economic impact in the U.S. of $40 billion!

Moreover, the annual economic impact of seasonal flu in the U.S. has been estimated at $87 billion. This estimate includes the cost of medical treatment for children which ranges from $300 to $4,000 per child per year, depending on whether hospitalization is required or only outpatient treatment. And when you consider that 5–20% of the population contracts the flu in any given year, these costs quickly add up.

The increased incidence of norovirus and *MRSA* also give rise for concern over the health and well-being of children. *Norovirus* alone is responsible for over 235,000 outpatient visits per year by children, 91,000 ER visits, and over 23,000 hospitalizations of children under the age of 18. In addition, *MRSA*, once restricted to the hospital environment, is now primarily transmitted in public gathering places, and is prevalent among children. To illustrate, between the years 2001–09 there was a 305% increase in the incidence of *MRSA* in children of 17 years or less. And the CDC reports that there has been a steady 10% per year increase in the incidence rate of children since then.

It is in this context that the value of cleaning in protecting the health of children and the general public can best be appreciated. Bottom line: a relatively modest investment in an effective cleaning and hygiene program can help avoid or significantly improve the quality of the indoor environment, protect public health, and reduce the social and economic impacts of infectious diseases.

Cleaning and Hygiene Reduce the Transmission of Infectious Diseases

To best appreciate how a cleaning and hygiene program can reduce the transmission of infectious diseases, it is important to first briefly explore how germs are spread.

For example, influenza and colds are primarily spread through large droplets that are produced when infected people cough, sneeze, or talk, sending the relatively large infectious droplets and very small sprays (aerosols) into the nearby air and into contact with other people. Large droplets can only travel a limited range; therefore, people should limit close contact (within 6 feet) with others when possible. In addition, the cold and flu are also spread by infected individuals touching objects such as doorknobs, elevator buttons, hand rails, and other frequently-touched surfaces, thus contaminating the object with viruses. The viruses are then transmitted to another person who touches the same object and then transfers the infected material from the hands to the nose, mouth, or eyes. That is why it is important to clean and disinfect frequently-touched surfaces.

Effective cleaning and disinfecting of environmental surfaces including "high touch" or frequently-touched surfaces (i.e., desks, countertops, faucet handles, doorknobs) significantly decreases the number of environmental pathogens including influenza and cold viruses on those surfaces or objects, which in turn reduces the risk of transmission and infection. Routine cleaning removes the soil and dirt that harbors the infectious agents, while disinfecting kills the remaining environmental pathogens.

Recommended Cleaning and Disinfection Practices to Prevent the Spread of Cold, Flu, and Other Infectious Diseases

The following cleaning and disinfection practices are recommended to help prevent the spread of influenza and cold viruses, and are largely based on the CDC recommendations which can be found at www.cdc.gov/flu/school/cleaning.htm.

While these CDC recommendations are targeted to schools, they are appropriate for day care, nurseries and other similar facilities.

1. Just clean. Do not underestimate the power of simply cleaning to reduce the risk of transmitting the influenza and cold viruses as well as other pathogens. Cleaning removes dirt, soil, and impurities that harbor germs and viruses like influenza and those that cause the common cold. Routine cleaning therefore plays a critical role in reducing the spread of flu and colds. Just as important, remember cleaning is often a necessary first step in disinfecting a surface, which actually kills the remaining germs.

2. Clean and disinfect frequently touched surfaces. Daily clean and disinfect surfaces and objects that are frequently touched, such as desks, countertops, doorknobs, and faucet handles. The frequency may be increased when there is a known outbreak. Immediately clean and disinfect surfaces that are visibly soiled with body fluids (vomit, urine, etc.) or blood. Follow precautions set forth in the OSHA Bloodborne Pathogen Standard to avoid contact with the fluid.

3. Simply do routine cleaning and disinfecting. It's important to match your cleaning and disinfecting activities to the types of germs you want to remove or kill. For example, most studies have shown that the flu virus can live and potentially infect a person for only 2 to 8 hours after being deposited on a surface. Therefore, it is not necessary to close facilities to clean or disinfect every surface in the building to slow the spread of flu.

4. Flu and cold viruses are relatively fragile. So standard or routine cleaning and disinfecting practices are sufficient to remove or kill them. Special cleaning and disinfecting processes, including wiping down walls and ceilings, or fumigating, are not necessary or recommended. These processes can irritate eyes, noses, throats, and skin; aggravate asthma; and cause other adverse side effects.

5. Clean and disinfect correctly. Always follow label directions on cleaning products and disinfectants. It is important to note that the directions on most disinfectant products require the surface to first be cleaned. First clean surfaces with a general-purpose cleaner to remove germs, and follow with an EPA-registered disinfectant to kill germs. Be sure to follow the label directions on the disinfectant for dwell time—the amount of time necessary for the disinfectant to reside on the surface in order to effectively kill the germs. Please be sure to make sure the surface remains wet during the dwell time to properly disinfect and kill the germs. Therefore, you may wish to select disinfectants that have shorter dwell times compared to other competing products.

6. Select EPA-registered products. When disinfecting frequently-touched surfaces, make certain to utilize EPA-approved disinfectants with label claims indicating that the product kills cold and flu viruses.

7. If a surface is not visibly dirty, you can clean it with an EPA-registered product that both cleans (removes soil and germs) and disinfects (kills germs) instead. Be sure to read the label directions carefully, as there may be a separate procedure for using the product as a cleaner or as a disinfectant.

8. Use disinfecting wipes on electronic items that are touched often, such as phones and computers. Pay close attention to the directions for using disinfecting wipes. It may be necessary to use more than one wipe to keep the surface wet for the stated length of contact time. Make sure that the electronics can withstand the use of liquids for cleaning and disinfecting.

9. Use products safely. Pay close attention to hazard warnings and directions on product labels and SDSs. Cleaning products and disinfectants may call for the use of gloves or eye protection. When appropriate, it is very important that such personal protective equipment be provided to employees.

10. Do not mix cleaners and disinfectants unless the labels clearly indicate that it is safe to do so. Combining certain products (such as chlorine bleach and cleaners containing ammonia) can result in serious injury or death.

11. Provide employee training. Ensure that custodial staff and others who use cleaners and disinfectants read and understand all instruction labels and understand the safe and appropriate use. Utilize the product Safety Data Sheet (SDS). Sometimes instructional materials and training will need to be provided in other languages.

12. Additional Resources. Please see the *Resources and Tools* section of this publication for additional information and programs that can help you effectively clean and disinfect to reduce the incidence of the flu and cold.

Hand Hygiene

Keeping hands clean is one of the most important steps we can take to avoid getting sick and spreading germs such as the influenza or cold virus to others. Many diseases and conditions are spread by not washing hands with soap and clean running water, or when not available, a hand sanitizer. For example, it is reported that handwashing:

- Reduces respiratory illnesses, like the flu and cold, in the general population by 21%
- Reduces the number of people who get sick with diarrhea by 31%
- Reduces diarrheal illness in people with weakened immune systems by 58%

Why Wash Hands. Handwashing with soap and clean running water removes germs from hands. This helps prevent infections from spreading because:

1. People frequently touch their eyes, nose, and mouth without even realizing it. Germs can get into the body through the eyes, nose, and mouth and make us sick.

2. Germs from unwashed hands can get into foods and drinks while people prepare or consume them. Germs can multiply in some types of foods or drinks, under certain conditions, and make people sick.

3. Germs from unwashed hands can be transferred to other objects such as handrails, table tops, or door knobs,

and then transferred to the hands of another person, who then becomes infected by touching his or her eyes, nose, or mouth.

4. Removing germs through handwashing therefore helps prevent the cold, flu, and other respiratory infections, diarrhea, and many other infectious diseases.

When You Should Wash Hands. Routine and frequent handwashing with running water and soap is important, and the CDC recommends that it be done:

1. After blowing your nose, coughing, sneezing.

2. After using the toilet.

3. Before and after preparing food.

4. Before you eat.

5. Before and after caring for someone who is sick.

6. After changing diapers or cleaning up a child who has used the toilet.

7. Before and after treating a cut or wound.

How to Wash Your Hands. While it is an activity that we are all familiar with, a recent study indicated that 95% of people observed washing their hands were doing it incorrectly. Therefore, it is worthwhile to re-examine the proper handwashing technique to ensure maximum removal of infectious agents.

1. Wet your hands with clean, running water (warm or cold), turn off the tap, and apply soap.

2. Lather your hands by rubbing them together with the soap. Be sure to lather the backs of your hands, between your fingers, and under your nails.

3. Scrub your hands for at least 20 seconds. Need a timer? Hum the "Happy Birthday" song from beginning to end twice.

4. Rinse your hands well under clean, running water.

5. Dry your hands using a clean towel or air dry them.

Hand Sanitizers. Washing hands with soap and water is the best way to reduce the number of microbes on them in most situations. However, if soap and water are not available, use an alcohol-based hand sanitizer. Alcohol-based hand sanitizers can quickly reduce the number of microbes on hands in some situations, but sanitizers do not eliminate all types of germs. It is important to note that hand sanitizers are not as effective when hands are visibly dirty.

Steps You Can Take to Reduce Exposure to the Cold, Flu and Other Infectious Diseases

In addition to implementing an effective cleaning and a hand hygiene program, there are a number of things you can do to reduce the transmission of the common cold and flu as well as other infectious diseases including, but not limited to, the following:

1. Encourage parents to keep sick children at home. That can be one of the best ways to prevent the spread of easily transmittable infections.

2. Provide resources and an environment that promotes personal hygiene. Provide tissues, no-touch trash cans, and hand soap for children and others to use.

3. Encourage children to wash their hands frequently with soap and water or with hand sanitizer if there is no soap or water available.

4. Encourage children to cover their coughs and sneezes with a tissue, or to cough and sneeze into their upper sleeves if tissues are not available. All children should wash their hands or use a hand sanitizer after they cough, sneeze, or blow their noses.

5. Promote healthy lifestyles, including good nutrition and exercise. A child's overall health impacts their body's immune system and can affect their ability to fight off, or recover from, an infectious disease.

Chapter 6

Passive Antimicrobial Solutions

Traditional surface cleaning and sanitizing methods have relied on a combination of application and abrading methods combined with liquid or soluble cleaning agents. In this chapter, we refer to these traditional methods as active cleaning solutions. Active cleaning solutions have proven to be very effective at disinfecting and sanitizing surfaces and rely on periodic execution of active cleaning protocols. Traditional active cleaning solutions do not protect surfaces from the reintroduction and propagation of bacterial, viral, and fungal microbes, which allow the possibility of contamination or infection prior to the execution of the next scheduled cleaning protocol. Additional risk of contamination and infection occur in the event of a breakdown in the cleaning schedule or execution of the cleaning protocol.

This chapter introduces the emerging technologies associated with self-sanitizing or self-disinfecting environmental surfaces or surface coatings that we categorically refer to as passive antimicrobial solutions. Since their commercialization in the early 1980s, passive antimicrobial solutions have progressively become more effective at reducing the presence of bacteria, viruses, and fungus. Passive antimicrobial solutions often utilize one of the following three technologies: ionic silver or copper nanoparticles – typically either embedded in solids, film coatings, or suspended in liquid solutions and applied as surface coatings; germicides such as Triclosan or quaternary ammonium chemical compounds – typically suspended in liquid resins or paints and applied as surface coatings; or photocatalytic nanoparticles (usually of titanium dioxide) – suspended in a water-based solution and applied by an electrostatic sprayer/mister.

There are quite a number of chemicals in other active and passive cleaners, disinfectants, and sanitizers that present varying degrees of health and safety concerns. Our readers can learn more about specific chemical concerns by referencing the Hazard Materials Information System product labeling guidelines and definitions which are a required section of the Safety Data Sheet of any chemical used in a product.

The history and technological advancement of passive antimicrobial solutions has largely been driven by the medical community, which has been concerned with the spread of illness between patients via facilities, equipment, and health care personnel. During the past 25 years, care providers and scientists have studied the persistence of targeted pathogens on environmental surfaces. There is conclusive evidence that *Methicillin Resistant Staphylococcus aureus (MRSA), Vancomycin Resistant Enterococcus species (VRE), Clostridium difficile (CDIF)* and *norovirus* can survive on surfaces for days and in certain environmental conditions for months. Furthermore, studies are connecting these conditions to patient-to-patient transmission of illness via the hands of healthcare personnel, equipment, and facilities of healthcare environments. Collectively these types of infection problems within health care are commonly referred to as nosocomial infections or sometimes Healthcare Acquired Infections (HAIs).

In an attempt to address these concerns, active cleaning and no-touch protocols have been introduced and refined for a number of years but have not always been found to be adequate in all circumstances. This has led to the consideration of passive antimicrobial solutions that continually work to reduce the presence of illness causing pathogens in healthcare environments. Most recently the healthcare community is generally investigating ionic metals, germicides, and photocatalytic coatings. To date, no findings have been published regarding the ability of these methods to decrease the incidence of healthcare–associated infections, although numerous studies are ongoing which focus on active and passive solutions and their interactions as well as clinical environments with variable pathogen challenges and conditions.

As clinical and applied research continues in healthcare, highly publicized bacterial and viral illness outbreaks in hospitality (most notably *norovirus* aboard cruise ships) and education in the late 1990s and growing in frequency and severity into the early 2000s have facilitated the introduction of passive antimicrobial solutions in these areas. This led to general preventative introductions of passive technologies in child-care, education, hospitality, business, and public sector facilities.

As passive antimicrobial solutions are being introduced into these various market segments, technologies are applied that target market specific concerns. In the following sections we will review a few product and technology examples in each market and how they are aligned to a specific set of concerns and needs.

Healthcare facility patients are typically immune-compromised and more susceptible to HAIs. In addition to continuing investment in sanitation protocols associated with healthcare instruments, passive technologies focus on healthcare personnel common touch points such as plastic equipment handles, keyboards, and furniture. Innovative companies such as **Microban**, who utilize the antimicrobial properties of silver ions, have forged meaningful and effective relationships with manufacturers to successfully embed **Microban** additives into common touch points of frequently handled equipment and furniture. More recently, the company **SealShield** has combined their silver ion antimicrobial-embedded technologies with waterproof computer keyboard and mouse designs to make products that are dishwasher safe. These products are cutting-edge examples of merging both active and passive antimicrobial technologies.

Child-care facilities have specific challenges with general hand hygiene and parental obligations which can result in sending sick children to child-care and drives a debate around participation. Education shares these concerns and has the additional concern of funding structures tied to a metric known as the Average Daily Attendance of students, which ties school district funding to each student attendance day. The biggest drivers of illness in child-care and education are influenza and outbreaks of *corona*, *rhino*, and *rota viruses* (respiratory and gastrointestinal viruses). There have also been significant outbreaks of *norovirus* within school districts.

Because so few viruses are required to result in a student falling ill and the illness is largely driven by viral infection, we are observing a hybrid approach being explored by daycare and school facilities. This hybrid model generally maintains traditional active cleaning protocols provided by cleaning personnel combined with increasing additions of passive antimicrobial solutions. The passive solutions can be divided into two categories. The first are toys and play structures. When it becomes necessary to replace these items, the replacements are increasingly made with materials and paints that are embedded with antimicrobials or with smooth finishes that improve the effectiveness of the active cleaning protocols. **PLAYTIME** is a good example of a company that provides soft play structures that utilize smooth finishes and antimicrobials to reduce the presence of bacteria and reduce fungal surface growth. The second passive category is coverings and coatings targeting common touch-points where viruses and bacteria can be spread through hand contact. The companies recognized that limited budgets prevent replacement of common touch-point fixtures with touchless options. Therefore, companies such as **SafeHandles** have produced low-cost coatings and coverings that when applied, reduce the presence of virus and bacteria on their surface, thus reducing the probability of microbial transmission by way of the common touch-point.

Child-care and educational environments present a unique challenge of poor hand-hygiene, common touch-points, child to child contact, and the inability of cleaning personnel to execute active cleaning protocols during daily child-care and school operations. While these facilities are actively cleaned after the daily operations conclude, pathogen introduction and propagation may occur by and between children during the course of a single day in these facilities. In recognizing these challenges, we are seeing proactive companies such as **SafeHandles**, **PLAYTIME**, and **SealShield** targeting common touch-points such as door handles, railings, play structures, and computer equipment to introduce their passive antimicrobial technologies.

As an example of specifically how these technologies work, we will take a closer look at **SafeHandles** whose products utilize innovative heat-shrink and adhesive application methods to cover door handles, push plates, and railings throughout a care or school facility. Once in place, **SafeHandles** constantly work to reduce the presence of illness causing pathogens on their surface that are introduced when touched by children.

Through this example, it becomes apparent how the passive antimicrobial solutions that these companies offer function to reduce child and staff exposure to illness-causing pathogens. These technologies also augment the effectiveness of nightly active cleaning protocols. Child-care and educational owners and administrators who understand these technologies can proactively work with their cleaning professionals to design and implement cleaning programs that increase attendance and participation by improving the health and well-being of both children and staff.

Outside of the healthcare and educational related markets, the largest concerns driving demand for passive antimicrobial solutions are productivity and identity. Productivity concerns are driven by labor statistics citing 69 million worker sick-days per year and average productivity losses of $1,685 per employee per year, which represent a significant impact to corporate bottom lines throughout the United States. However, business efforts as of this writing have not extended beyond the use of active cleaning services and alcohol-based hand sanitizers, such as the ubiquitous **Purell** dispensers, placed in selected locations throughout businesses. The cruise line industry is a notable exception, as it has had to address customer and regulatory concerns associated with highly publicized outbreaks of norovirus aboard cruise ships. Industry leaders are actively testing rigorous disinfecting and sanitizing cleaning protocols and driving further investment into innovative water-based coatings that contain suspended titanium-oxide nanoparticles. These ultrathin coatings create a photocatalytic surface whose oxidative properties breakdown organics on the coating's surface which include fungus, bacteria, and viruses. While commercial availability of these technologies is limited and costs are high, considerable investment is being made to gain regulatory approval through the Environmental Protection Agency (EPA), which is essential to the eventual commercialization of these technologies.

References

Bright, R. Kelly, PhD, Boone, A. Stephanie, MPH, PhD, Gerba, P. Charles, Ph.D. (2009). Occurrence of bacteria and viruses on elementary classroom surfaces and the potential role of classroom hygiene in the spread of infectious diseases. The Journal of School Nursing.

Carling, C. Phillip, M.D., Bartley, M. Judene, MS/MPH/CIC (2010). Evaluating hygienic cleaning in health care settings: What you do not know can harm you patients. American Journal of Infection Control.

Gwaltney, M. Jack Dr, Hendley, J. Owen (1982). Transmission of experimental rhinovirus infection by contaminated surfaces. American Journal of Epidemiology.

Lam, L. Wanda (2000). Antimicrobial effect of Triclosan-impregnated hospital furniture surfaces. Kalamazoo College Health Sciences Thesis Collection.

Satter, A. Syed, PhD (2010). Promises and pitfalls of recent advances in chemical means of preventing the spread of nosocomial infections by environmental surfaces. American Journal of Infection Control.

Tamimi, H. Akrum, PhD, Carlino, Sheri BS, Gerba P. Charles Ph.D. (2014). Long-term efficacy of a self-disinfecting coating in an intensive care unit. Elsevier.

Weber, J. David, M.D. /MPH (2012). Self-disinfecting surfaces: Review of current methodologies and future prospects. American Journal of Infection Control.

Shapiro, D. Eugene (1984). Exclusion of ill children for day-care center. Clinical Pediatrics.

Chapter 7

Resources and Tools

There are increasing scientific, consumer, and government concerns about toxic chemicals in everyday products. This increasing attention to chemical toxicity is resulting in significant research, evaluation, and adoption of safer chemicals, materials, and products. Where safer effective alternatives are not currently available, efforts are underway in many sectors to develop them. The chemical product value chain (from chemical manufacturer, to formulator, brand, and retailer) is increasingly collaborating to identify needs for safer alternatives and ways to encourage their development and adoption in the marketplace.

Organizations such as the <u>Green Chemistry and Commerce Council (GC3)</u>[21], a business-to-business forum dedicated to accelerating green chemistry across supply chains and sectors, are working to identify barriers to greener, more sustainable chemicals and products, and to develop partnerships to overcome them. A number of efforts are engaging institutional purchasers to support them in their efforts to accelerate sustainable products.

Nonetheless, purchasing safer, sustainable, and effective products can be a challenge for purchaser. Many resources, however, are available to help purchasers understand chemical hazards and the availability of safer products and how to buy them. Below is a listing of some of these resources. Those making purchasing policies or decisions should talk to their peers, trade associations, government environmental and health agencies, local public health and environmental organizations, university researchers, and others to find the right kind of information and assistance to meet their needs.

Sources of Information on Hazardous Substances and Safer Alternatives

- California Prop 65[22]

Prop 65 is California's law to protect the state's drinking-water sources from being contaminated with chemicals known to cause cancer, birth defects, or other reproductive harm. The state keeps an updated list of chemicals that trigger a warning on products because of these hazards.

- California Safer Consumer Products[23]

The Safer Consumer Products program strives to reduce toxic chemicals in products consumers buy and use. It identifies specific products containing potentially harmful chemicals and asks manufacturers to answer two questions: 1) Is this chemical necessary? 2) Is there a safer alternative? The site links to the program's list of chemicals of concern, as well as priority products where those chemicals may be found.

- ChemHAT – Chemical Hazard and Alternatives Toolbox[24]

ChemHAT is a database where users can search for hazard information on chemicals based on authoritative lists of chemicals. ChemHAT was created to answer two questions: "Can this chemical in my workplace affect my health?" and "Are there safer alternatives?"

- Green Science Policy Institute[25]

The Green Science Policy Institute's mission is to facilitate responsible use of chemicals to protect human and ecological health. The Institute educates and builds partnerships among scientists, regulators, businesses, and public-interest groups to develop innovative solutions for reducing harmful chemicals in products. The Institute is working with institutional purchasers to substitute six classes[26] of chemicals of concern in products, including highly fluorinated chemicals, anti-microbials, flame retardants, bisphenols and phthalates, organic solvents, and certain metals.

- Hazardous Substances Databank (HSDB)[27]

HSDB is a toxicology database on the National Library of Medicine's[28] (NLM Toxicology Data Network[29] (TOXNET®). It focuses on the toxicology of potentially hazardous chemicals. It contains information on human exposure, industrial hygiene, emergency handling procedures, environmental fate, regulatory requirements, nanomaterials, and related areas. HSDB is produced by the National Library of Medicine, part of the National Institutes of Health.

- Health Care Without Harm[30]

Health Care Without Harm is a global network of health professionals, community groups, health-affected constituencies, and others that maintains information on chemicals of concern in the health care sector, as well as available alternatives.

- Interstate Clearinghouse on Chemicals[31]

The Interstate Clearinghouse on Chemicals (IC2) is an association of state, local, and tribal governments that promotes a clean environment, healthy communities, and a vital economy through the development and use of safer chemicals and products. The IC2 hosts a list of chemicals of concern in various states, evaluations of alternatives, and a database of state chemicals policies.

- Occupational Safety and Health Administration – Transitioning to Safer Chemicals Toolkit[32]

OSHA has developed this step-by-step toolkit to provide employers and workers with information, methods, tools, and guidance on using informed substitution in the workplace. The toolkit provides case studies and links to assist firms and others in transitioning to safer chemicals.

- OECD Alternatives Assessment Tool Selector[33]

The OECD Substitution and Alternatives Assessment Toolbox (SAAT) is a compilation of resources relevant to chemical substitution and alternatives assessments, including lists of chemicals of concern, tools for evaluating alternatives, and case examples.

- SUBSPORT – Substitution Support Portal[34]

SUBSPORT is a multilingual platform for information exchange on alternative substances and technologies, as well as tools and guidance for substance evaluation and substitution management. The SUBSPORT portal contains lists of chemicals of concern, case studies, and tools for evaluating chemical hazards and alternatives.

- Toxics Use Reduction Institute, UMass Lowell[35]

The Massachusetts Toxics Use Reduction Act establishes a Toxic or Hazardous Substance list and information about chemical hazards for substances covered under the Act. The Toxics Use Reduction Institute (TURI) at the University of Massachusetts Lowell provides resources and tools to reduce or substitute substances covered under the act.

- U.S. Environmental Protection Agency – ChemView[36]

EPA's ChemView database combines information on chemical hazards and safer alternatives from multiple sources into a single searchable interface. The site contains information EPA receives and develops about chemicals including those on EPA's Safer Chemical Ingredient List.

Information on Sustainable Purchasing Guidelines and Specifications

- Responsible Purchasing Network[37]

RPN is a non-profit international network of buyers that has developed a wide array of resources that can make it easier for institutional purchasers to identify, specify, and buy low-toxicity goods and services. This includes purchasing guides that recommend specifications and procurement strategies for specific product categories, such as low-emitting furniture, low-toxicity architectural and traffic paint, low-mercury lighting equipment, and safer alternatives to polystyrene foodservice ware. RPN's website and webinars also highlight certifications—and cooperative purchasing opportunities—for low-toxicity products such as cleaners, hand soaps, floor maintenance chemicals, office supplies, and more.

- Sustainable Purchasing Leadership Council[38]

The SPLC is a non-profit organization whose mission is to support and recognize purchasing leadership that accelerates the transition to a prosperous and sustainable future. The Council's *Guidance for Leadership in Sustainable Purchasing Version 1.0* is a handbook for strategic sustainable purchasing and serves as the basis for a future *Rating System for Leadership in Sustainable Purchasing* that rewards organizations that demonstrate leadership in sustainable purchasing.

Information to Help Understand Ecolabels and Standards

- Challenge the Label[39]

The site describes what sustainability claims are and how to determine if a sustainability claim is credible. It is part of the ISEAL Alliance[40], a non-governmental organization whose mission is to strengthen sustainability standards systems for the benefit of people and the environment.

- Environmental Protection Agency (EPA) Greener Products Portal[41]

The EPA Greener Products Portal is designed to help the user navigate the increasingly important and complex world of greener products. It allows users to search for EPA programs related to greener products based on the type of user and his or her specific product interests. It also links to additional greener products information from EPA and other sources, and includes an introduction to ecolabels and standards.

Independent Third Party Ecolabels

- Green Seal[42]

Green Seal develops lifecycle-based sustainability standards for products, services, and companies and offers third-party certification for those that meet the criteria in the standard. Product categories include household products, construction materials and equipment, paints and coatings, printing and writing paper, cleaning products, and more.

- Cradle to Cradle Certified Product Standard[43]

The Cradle to Cradle Products Innovation Institute administers the Cradle to Cradle Certified Product Standard, which provides designers and manufacturers with criteria and requirements for continually improving what products are made of and how they are made. Categories include apparel, shoes, and accessories, home and office supply, interior design and furniture, and more

- Green Good Housekeeping Seal[44]

The Good Housekeeping Institute (GHI) reviews and verifies a range of data related to the product's measurable environmental impact for its *Green Good Housekeeping Seal*. Reduction of water and energy use in manufacturing and product usage, ingredient, and product safety; reduction in packaging; and the brand's corporate social responsibility are among factors considered. Categories include cleaning products, beauty products, paints and coatings, appliances and electronics, paper goods, building products, and food and beverages.

- GreenGuard and EcoLogo[45]

Underwriters Laboratory is the exclusive provider of GREENGUARD Certification for products that meet stringent chemical emissions requirements, and ECOLOGO Certification for products that meet multi-attribute, lifecycle-based sustainability standards.

- Safer Choice[46]

The U.S. Environmental Protection Agency administers the Safer Choice program (formerly Design for Environment, DfE), a label that covers over 2,000 products. In addition to safer ingredients, Safer Choice includes requirements for performance, packaging, pH, and volatile organic compounds.

Tools for Evaluating Chemical Hazards in Products and Safer Alternatives

- WERCSmart,[47] GreenWercs,[48] and Good Guide[49]

UL Environment has these three tools to help understand and assess product ingredients. WERCSmart and GreenWercs collect data from product suppliers that can be used by purchasers to identify and screen out chemicals of concern. GoodGuide evaluates products for health, environmental, and social issues, and provides a summary score and detailed ratings. GoodGuide rates over 250,000 products. Purchaser preferences can be prioritized.

- Material IQ[50]

Developed by the non-profit Green Blue Institute, MiQ provides third-party-validated toxicity data and information about other sustainability attributes to end-users and purchasers.

- GreenScreen for Safer Chemicals[51]

GreenScreen for Safer Chemicals is a method of comparative Chemical Hazard Assessment (CHA) that can be used for identifying chemicals of high concern and safer alternatives.

GreenScreen was developed and is a project of Clean Production Action.

- CleanGredients[52]

CleanGredients is an online database of chemical products (a.k.a. "ingredients") used primarily to formulate residential, institutional, industrial, and janitorial cleaning products that have been preapproved to meet the U.S. EPA's Safer Choice Standard.

Reports and Resources on
Green Cleaning and Disinfection

UCSF Institute for Health & Aging, UC Berkeley Center for Environmental Research and Children's Health, Informed Green Solutions, and California Department of Pesticide Regulation. *A Green Cleaning, Sanitizing, and Disinfecting: Toolkit for Early Care and Education*, University of California, San Francisco School of Nursing: San Francisco, California, 2013. Accessible at:

http://www2.epa.gov/sites/production/files/documents/ece_curriculumfinal.pdf

Green Schools Initiative and Green Purchasing Institute. *Use Safer Disinfectants and Disinfecting Practices.* Accessible at:

http://www.greenschools.net/article.php?id=278

Healthy Schools Network, *Guide to Green Cleaning, 2011.* Accessible at:

http://www.healthyschools.org/downloads/Guide_to_Green_Cleaning_2011.pdf

Healthy Schools Network, *Sanitizers and Disinfectants Guide. 2014.* Accessible at:

http://www.cleaningforhealthyschools.org/documents/Sanitizers_and_Disinfectants_2014.pdf

Healthy Schools Network, et al. *Green Cleaning / Healthy Products Toolkit.* Accessible at:

http://www.cleaningforhealthyschools.org/

Responsible Purchasing Network. *Green Cleaning Purchasing Guide.* Accessible at:

http://www.responsiblepurchasing.org/purchasing_guides/cleaners/index.php

U.S. Environmental Protection Agency. *Environmentally Preferable Purchasing, Cleaning.* Accessible at:

http://www.epa.gov/epp/pubs/products/cleaning.htm

National Cleaning for Healthier Schools and Infection Control Workgroup. *Cleaning for Healthier Schools – Infection Control Handbook, 2010.* Accessible at:

http://www.informedgreensolutions.org/?q=publications/cleaning-healthier-schools-infection-control-handbook

Notes, Chapter 7

[21]www.greenchemistryandcommerce.org
[22] http://oehha.ca.gov/prop65/prop65_list/Newlist.html
[23] http://www.dtsc.ca.gov/SCP/index.cfm
[24]http://www.chemhat.org/
[25] http://greensciencepolicy.org/
[26] http://www.sixclasses.org/
[27]http://www.nlm.nih.gov/pubs/factsheets/hsdbfs.html
[28] http://www.nlm.nih.gov/nlmhome.html
[29]http://toxnet.nlm.nih.gov/
[30] https://noharm.org/
[31]http://www.theic2.org/chemicals-concern
[32]https://www.osha.gov/dsg/safer_chemicals/index.html
[33]http://www.oecdsaatoolbox.org/
[34]http://www.subsport.eu/
[35]http://www.turi.org/
[36]http://www.epa.gov/oppt/existingchemicals/pubs/chemview
[37]http://www.responsiblepurchasing.org/
[38]https://www.sustainablepurchasing.org/
[39]http://www.challengethelabel.org/
[40]http://www.isealalliance.org/

[41]http://www.epa.gov/greenerproducts/index.html
[42]http://www.greenseal.org/
[43]http://www.c2ccertified.org/
[44]http://www.goodhousekeeping.com/institute/about-the-institute/a17832/about-green-good-housekeeping-seal/
[45]http://industries.ul.com/environment
[46]http://www2.epa.gov/saferchoice
[47]http://www.thewercs.com/products-and-services/wercsmart-retail
[48]http://www.thewercs.com/products-and-services/greenwercs
[49]http://www.goodguide.com/about/ratings
[50]http://www.materialiq.com/
[51]http://www.greenscreenchemicals.org/
[52]http://www.cleangredients.org/about/

Appendix

Christ Supplies offers a number of products that can help child-care facilities create a safer and more enjoyable environment for children. Among those are:

Disinfectants / Sanitizers

Beyond Green Cleaning Disinfectant Cleaner

[EPA Toxicity Category 4]

PURE Hard Surface Disinfectant

[EPA Toxicity Category 4]

Sani-Spray Sanitizing Tablets

[EPA Toxicity Category 2]

Environmentally Preferable Cleaners

Alpha Chemical Services Items
[Northeast & East Coast]

PDQ Manufacturing Products
[Southeast customers]

Seatex Corporation Products
[Southwest customers]

Floor Mats

Guardian Anti-Drug and Daycare mats

Guardian Ecoguard mats (made from recycled drinking bottles)

Passive Antimicrobial Products

SafeHandles (shrink sleeves and roll tape for door and faucet handles)

Toys

Green Toys (manufactured from recycled plastic milk containers)

Pedal Cars and Scoot-A-Long Cars

PLAYTIME play area elements

For more information about any of these products, please visit our website: **www.christ-supplies.com**

Or you may call us at these telephone numbers:

Nashville Office (order inquiries)
(888) 852–6848

New Orleans Office (sales information)
(504) 289–8622

Houston Office (technical information)
(281) 773–0778